THE COMPLETE FIGHTER DIET FOR BEGINNERS

Shed Fat, Build Strong Muscles, Control Your Appetite, and Unleash the Champion Within You

Chris Preston, RDN

ACKNOWLEDGEMENTS

I would like to express my deepest gratitude to everyone who supported me throughout the journey of creating this book. To my family and friends, your unwavering encouragement and patience have been invaluable.

A special thanks to my team, whose expertise and guidance were crucial in developing the dietary plans and recipes shared in this book. Your insights have been a cornerstone of this work.

I am also deeply grateful to my editor, Michael Jones, for your meticulous attention to detail and for helping shape this book into a comprehensive and accessible guide.

To the support groups and communities who shared their experiences and provided feedback, your contributions have enriched this book and made it more relatable for those living with fructose intolerance.

Lastly, to my readers, thank you for embarking on this journey with me. I hope this book provides you with the knowledge and tools to navigate your dietary needs and improve your quality of life.

COPYRIGHT

This book is intended to provide general information about diet and nutrition. It is not intended as a substitute for professional medical advice, diagnosis, or treatment. Always seek the advice of your physician or other qualified health provider with any questions you may have regarding a medical condition.

TABLE OF CONTENTS

INTRODUCTION

When it comes to specific eating plans designed to boost athletic performance, the Fighter Diet stands out as an exceptionally well-thought-out plan. This food plan goes above and beyond what is typically considered "sports nutrition" and is designed for people who are really dedicated to their training and want to perform at their highest level.

In order to meet the demands of strenuous physical exercise, the Fighter Diet places an emphasis on a well-balanced macronutrient profile. The unique thing about it is how these macronutrient ratios are carefully adjusted during different training cycles. This helps to match the body's nutritional needs with its ever-changing demands.

In addition to macronutrients, the Fighter Diet prioritizes micronutrient density by combining a wide variety of whole food antioxidants, vitamins, and minerals to promote overall health.

A sustainable option for those committed to reaching and sustaining peak physical performance, the Fighter Diet stands out due to its versatility, which accommodates varied dietary choices and lifestyles. To put it simply, the Fighter

Diet is a professional-level eating plan that has

been painstakingly crafted for those who want to

be physically and mentally fit for life.

PART I

UNDERSTANDING THE SCIENCE BEHIND THE FIGHTER DIET

People who exercise at a high intensity, like those who do martial arts or combat sports, might benefit from following the Fighter Diet, a dietary plan that promotes peak performance and health. This eating plan is based on the tenets of sports nutrition and is designed to supply the energy, nutrients, and fat that athletes need to perform at their best for longer periods of time.

The Fighter Diet revolves around a balanced distribution of macronutrients, with an emphasis on the relative significance of carbs, proteins, and fats. Fueling strenuous workouts and keeping muscular glycogen reserves full are two of the most important functions of carbohydrates. Preferably consumed throughout the day are high-quality, complex carbs including fruits, vegetables, whole grains, and other carbs.

The Fighter Diet places a premium on protein because of the critical function it plays in facilitating muscle development and repair. In order to meet the demands of intense exercise, recover quickly, and avoid muscle breakdown, it is important to consume enough protein. To fulfill the nutritional requirements of combatants without needless calorie excess, lean protein sources such chicken, fish, lean meats, and plant-based alternatives are included.

One of the most important parts of the Fighter Diet is eating healthy fats. Essential fatty acids, including omega-3 and omega-6, help keep hormone levels stable, promote healthy joints, and add to general well-being. For a balanced diet, incorporate foods like avocados, almonds, seeds, and fatty fish, which are good sources of fat.

Essential tenets of the Fighter Diet include controlling portion sizes and timing meals. To maximize performance and recuperation, it is helpful to organize meals strategically around training sessions. While carbohydrate and protein-based post-workout diet aims to restore glycogen reserves and facilitate muscle regeneration, energy-rich pre-training meals are more concerned with supplying easily accessible energy.

In order to avoid dehydration and keep performance high, the Fighter Diet makes sure that you drink enough of water. Combatants should drink water regularly throughout the day and pay specific attention to their electrolyte balance before, during, and after strenuous exercise.

As a means to address possible nutritional deficiencies and boost performance, supplements are taken into account within the Fighter Diet framework. The focus, though, is on getting those nutrients from whole foods whenever you can.

Athletes that participate in high-intensity exercise can benefit greatly from the Fighter Diet, a holistic approach to nutrition that emphasizes timing, hydration, and balanced macronutrients. Based on sound scientific research, this diet plan is designed to meet the rigorous nutritional requirements of combat sports, helping athletes reach their full potential without sacrificing their health in the process.

Understanding the Fighter Diet Philosophy

The Fighter Diet, developed by Pauline Nordin, is an all-encompassing way of eating and living that helps those who train very physically, especially those who participate in combat sports and strength training, perform better and look better. This ideology is based on a thorough comprehension of the specific dietary requirements of athletes as well as on scientific concepts and real-world experience.

A key principle of the Fighter Diet is the consumption of entire foods that are rich in nutrients. In order to foster muscle growth, increase energy, and improve general health, the dietary framework recommends that people primarily consume lean proteins, complex carbs, and necessary fats. The goal of this strategy is to provide athletes with a complete set of micronutrients, vitamins, and minerals so they can train and recuperate at their best.

An important part of the Fighter Diet concept is controlling calories. Keeping a sustainable energy balance that corresponds with individual exercise needs is more important than strictly following to calorie tracking. This method seeks to minimize calorie surpluses that might cause undesirable fat growth and excessive caloric deficits that can damage muscle development and impede athletic progress.

The Fighter Diet is also known for its cyclical carbohydrate consumption. To maximize glycogen store, insulin sensitivity, and fat utilization for energy, the diet deliberately incorporates low-carbohydrate days during rest or less active phases and high-carbohydrate days during hard training times.

Furthermore, the Fighter Diet acknowledges that staying hydrated is crucial for optimal physical performance. It is recommended to drink enough of water in order to improve metabolic function, nutritional absorption, and digestion. An important part of getting back on your feet and staying in top shape is making sure you drink enough of water.

The Fighter Diet isn't only about food; it's also about other aspects of your lifestyle, including getting enough sleep, handling stress, and taking supplements. In order to recuperate and maintain hormonal balance, getting enough quality sleep is essential. To lessen the detrimental effects of chronic stress on performance, it is recommended to practice effective stress management techniques. In order to improve general health and prevent nutritional deficiencies, personalized supplementing plans are put in place.

The Fighter Diet is a science-based, all-encompassing way of eating and living that caters to the special needs of athletes who are constantly pushing themselves to their physical limits. The Fighter Diet is a program that promotes peak performance, resilience, and a toned body by focusing on nutrient-dense meals, controlling calorie consumption, optimizing carbohydrate cycling, keeping hydrated, and addressing lifestyle issues.

Unveiling the Fundamentals of Nutrition for Fighters

A fighter's diet is built on a solid foundation of nutrition knowledge, carefully designed to enhance performance, stamina, and recuperation. Fighters' specific meal plans are more than just a habit; they're strategic blueprints for meeting the high energy needs of their training and competing at a high level. By delving into the essentials of the fighter's diet, we can see how this nutritional framework is built.

A fighter's diet relies on a balanced macronutrient distribution. Sustained performance requires an energy balance that is shaped by the triad of carbohydrates, proteins, and lipids. To ensure glycogen reserves are sufficiently restocked for high-intensity exercises and contests, carbohydrates serve as the principal fuel source. Proteins, on the other hand, are essential for building and repairing muscles, since they supply the amino acids needed to maintain the fighter's body. Simultaneously, high-quality fats promote general well-being and serve as an additional source of energy during extended physical activity.

An athlete's caloric intake must precisely correspond to their energy expenditure while training. Maintaining weight class standards while feeding strenuous exercises is a well crafted skill. Knowing the fighter's unique metabolic rate, training intensity, and objectives is crucial for this. Without a question, a fighter's diet is not a cookie-cutter method, but rather a tailored and flexible plan that changes over time to meet the demands of the fighter.

Micronutrients, which are sometimes overlooked despite their critical relevance, are vital to the fighter's general well-being and efficiency. The immune system, bone density, and metabolic rate can all benefit from a diet rich in vitamins and minerals. In order to provide complete and holistic nutritional support, the fighter's diet equally prioritizes macronutrient-rich meals as micronutrient-rich ones.

An essential part of any fighter's diet is staying hydrated. Impaired cognitive function, reduced endurance, and compromised recovery can result from dehydration. Optimal hydration, taking into account both personal requirements and external factors, is crucial for sustained peak performance. Strategic hydration is an important part of a fighter's dietary routine since electrolytes are lost through perspiration during strenuous training sessions.

The fighter's diet is a well-coordinated composition of water, micronutrients, and macronutrients. Fighters may accomplish the strenuous physical demands of their profession with the help of this adaptable and individualized eating plan, which guarantees that they will enter the ring or cage in peak physical condition.

Metabolic Optimization: Key Principles for Peak Performance

A fighter's diet becomes an important consideration in the quest for optimal performance in the demanding realm of combat sports, which is closely related to the optimization of metabolic processes. This important part of training for sports calls for a sophisticated grasp of fundamental concepts that extend beyond basic nutrition and into the complexities of metabolic efficiency.

Thoughtful study of macronutrient distribution is essential for a fighter's metabolic optimization diet. The foundation of this eating plan is finding the right mix of carbs, proteins, and fats. Carbohydrates are essential for maintaining endurance and power production, and they are also the main source of energy during intense training sessions. To back up the physical demands of intense combat training, proteins are also essential for muscle development and repair. To further aid in maintaining energy levels and metabolic health, healthy fats should be purposefully included.

An other crucial component of the fighter's metabolic optimization system is timing. In order to maximize the body's potential, it is crucial to strategically coordinate dietary consumption with exercise sessions. Before training, eat something balanced to fill up your energy reservoir, and after your workout, eat something to help your muscles recover and glycogen reserves refill. Sustaining energy levels and promoting adequate metabolic adaptability are both achieved through the careful orchestration of food timing.

An often-overlooked but crucial component of the fighter's metabolic equation is hydration. Overall metabolic efficiency, recuperation time, and performance can all take a hit when you're dehydrated. An essential part of any fighter's nutrition plan should be getting enough water, with the amount consumed depending on the individual's demands and the intensity of their training.

On top of that, optimizing metabolic rate should revolve around micronutrient density. Enzymatic activities, energy metabolism, and general physiological health all rely on essential vitamins and minerals. A well-rounded diet rich in fruits, vegetables, and whole foods promotes a strong and efficient metabolism by providing a wide range of micronutrients.

Ultimately, there are many moving parts to a fighter's diet that should be optimized for metabolic tasks. In order to reach and maintain optimum performance in combat sports, athletes must pay close attention to the timing, micronutrient density, macronutrient distribution, and hydration of their meals.

Navigating the Journey to Optimal Physical Performance

Achieving peak physical performance calls for a methodical strategy, and the Fighter Diet is an intimidating companion on this life-altering path. Getting in the best shape of your life is no easy feat; it requires a balanced approach to food, exercise, and mental toughness. Accuracy becomes our guide as we follow the Fighter Diet to discover our latent abilities along this complex path.

The Fighter Diet is based on a strategic framework for nutrition. In order to achieve peak performance, it is essential to fuel the body with a balanced combination of macro and micronutrients. To fuel the rigorous training that fighters undergo, this diet places an emphasis on lean proteins, complex carbs, and necessary fats. With every mouthful, you're consciously strengthening your body's capacity to survive and thrive.

A regiment tailored to combatants is an adjunct to the nutritional base. A combat athlete's body is a well-tuned machine that needs a wide variety of activities to develop strength, speed, and stamina; this is acknowledged by the Fighter Diet. A symphony of motions designed to increase strength and accuracy, the program includes everything from skill-specific drills to high-intensity interval training. Fitness is considerably more than just being in shape; it's about molding a body to handle the stresses of the ring or octagon with ease.

The path to peak physical performance, however, goes beyond the concrete domains of diet and exercise. The Fighter Diet recognizes the importance of mental toughness as a foundational quality for reaching one's full potential. Mindfulness exercises and mental conditioning are the cornerstones of the diet, which helps its adherents overcome anxiety, maintain concentration under duress, and develop the unwavering resolve that characterizes a champion.

With this all-encompassing strategy, the Fighter Diet is like a trusted friend in the never-ending quest for greatness. It turns the journey to peak physical performance into an intentional, strategic journey, where every step is a calculated move towards becoming more powerful, agile, and resilient. Along the way, the Fighter Diet is a trusted companion that helps people reach their peak physical performance.

PART II

BUILDING THE FOUNDATION: MACRONUTRIENTS UNVEILED

Knowing the ins and outs of macronutrients is critical for peak athletic performance and general well-being. Carbohydrates, proteins, and fats are the cornerstones of the fighter diet; they're crucial for fuelling the body, promoting muscle building, and improving recovery.

Combat athletes who want to maintain high-intensity exercises and rigorous training sessions must consume carbohydrates, frequently referred to as the body's principal energy source. You may stay active for longer with the help of complex carbs, which are present in fruits, vegetables, whole grains, and other plant-based foods. Maintaining a steady intake of refined carbs is essential for optimal performance since they cause energy spikes and crashes if consumed in excess.

An essential component of any fighter's diet for repairing and growing muscle is protein. After a workout, your body needs time to heal and repair, and getting the right amount of protein can assist with that. Fighters may fulfill their nutritional needs while keeping their diets interesting by eating a variety of protein sources, including lean meats, poultry, fish, eggs, and plant-based alternatives like beans and tofu.

Fats, contrary to popular belief, are essential for maintaining energy levels and general health. Consuming healthy fats from foods such as nuts, seeds, avocados, and olive oil can help regulate hormones and improve the absorption of vitamins that are fat-soluble. Maintaining a healthy diet of both saturated and unsaturated fats is crucial for optimal brain function and sustained energy during moderate exercise.

The key to unlocking optimal physical performance in the rigorous pursuit of a fighter's diet is understanding the intricate interplay between carbs, proteins, and lipids. In combat sports, a sustainable and successful diet is built around an ever-evolving process of tailoring macronutrient consumption to individual needs and training demands.

Precision Nutrition: Micronutrients for Fighters

To reach one's full potential in the cutthroat realm of elite combat sports, one must do more than just train hard and get in shape. In order to meet the specific requirements of fighters, a well-thought-out diet plan is crucial, with an emphasis on micronutrients. In this post, we'll look at the importance of fighters' precise nutrition and how micronutrients are crucial to their health and success on the mat.

Supplementing a fighter's diet with micronutrients like vitamins is essential. In order to keep energy levels up and the immune system strong, it is vital to consume these micronutrients in a balanced diet. For example, vitamin A is essential for good eyesight and immune system function, vitamin C helps make collagen and is a powerful antioxidant, so it can fight against the oxidative damage that comes with rigorous exercise.

Equally important for combatants are minerals, which contribute to a variety of physiological processes. Because of the extreme physical demands placed on combat athletes, it is crucial that they take calcium and magnesium supplements to maintain healthy bones and muscles. In order to maintain endurance and general performance during training and competition, iron—another vital mineral—is required for oxygen transport in the blood.

Fighters who want to maximize their cardiovascular health and manage inflammation must have omega-3 fatty acids, which are necessary lipids. Fish oil, chia seeds, and flaxseeds are good sources of these fats, which help athletes heal faster and have less inflammation, so they can stay in top physical shape.

A fighter's dietary regimen would be incomplete without enough hydration, as it affects both performance and recuperation. When it comes to nerve impulses, muscular contractions, and fluid equilibrium, electrolytes like chloride, potassium, and sodium are crucial. Hydration is an important part of many combat sports since it improves physical performance and helps with weight control.

Precision nutrition for athletes goes beyond only looking at macronutrients; it highlights the importance of micronutrients for maintaining health and performance. For fighters aiming to thrive in the intense and competitive world of combat sports, it is crucial to have a balanced diet rich in vitamins, minerals, vital fats, and water.

The Role of Vitamins in Immune Support and Recovery

The importance of vitamins in combat training and high-performance sports for improving immunity and speeding recovery is immense. An crucial component of a fighter's diet that enhances the athlete's capacity to endure intensive training and competition is the addition of certain micronutrients. In the context of a fighter's dietary plan, this exploration digs into the multifaceted function of vitamins, specifically their influence on immunological resilience and post-exertional recovery.

Vitamin C, well-known for its ability to strengthen the immune system, is an essential component of this dietary strategy. This vitamin, which is water-soluble and found in a wide variety of fruits and vegetables, is an effective weapon in the fight against disease. In addition to scavenging free radicals, its antioxidant capabilities are crucial for bolstering the immune system's defenses against outside invaders. Because of the increased stress that comes with fighting, it is crucial for fighters to consume plenty of vitamin C.

The immune system's toolbox must also include vitamin D, often known as the "sunshine vitamin." It is well-known that vitamin D helps bones, but less is known about the impact it has on the immune system. There is evidence that it helps with immune response modulation and inflammation reduction, two crucial aspects of an athlete's road to recovery. Boosting the fighter's immunity and general well-being is possible via getting enough sun exposure or eating vitamin D-rich meals.

The B-vitamin complex, which includes B6, B9 (folate), and B12, is another set of three crucial micronutrients that are important for the immune system and healing. These vitamins are involved in several processes, including energy metabolism, DNA synthesis, and immune cell formation. Athletes who want to perform at their best in the brutal world of combat sports strategically choose to take B-vitamins since they help with recuperation and energy levels.

When it comes to a fighter's diet, the careful addition of vitamins goes beyond just basic nourishment. It develops into a sophisticated plan to boost immunity and speed up recuperation, two things that are crucial for long-term success in the game. Vitamins C, D, and the B-complex each play unique functions, and fighters may get a nutritional advantage beyond just fuel by understanding these responsibilities. This can help them be more resilient and thrive in their athletic endeavors.

Adapting the Diet to Training Cycles and Fight Preparation

It takes a methodical strategy to training, recuperation, and nutrition to reach one's full potential in the world of combat sports; natural ability isn't enough. Tuning one's diet to different training cycles and phases of fight preparation is crucial for long-term success as a fighter, as it optimizes one's physical and mental skills.

Building a strong nutritional base should be prioritized in the early phases of a training cycle. Having a balanced diet that includes enough of protein, carbs, and healthy fats is key to this. Consuming enough protein aids in muscle repair and development, while carbs supply the fuel for strenuous workouts. For optimum hormone synthesis and metabolic efficiency in general, it is necessary to include vital fats.

The fighter's diet needs to be carefully modified to suit the increased energy demands of training as the intensity of training increases in the middle period of preparation. To restore glycogen levels that are lost after intense exercises, carbohydrate consumption becomes increasingly important. Consuming complex carbs during training sessions is a great way to fuel performance and speed up recovery, therefore timing is crucial. Dehydration can reduce mental and physical performance, therefore being properly hydrated is also crucial.

In order to be in the best possible shape for the big day, a well-planned nutritional plan is essential as fight training nears its end. When trying to lose weight, it's important to watch your calorie consumption while still getting all the nutrients your body needs. Maintaining a high protein diet helps maintain muscle mass, while controlling carbohydrate and water consumption helps reach weight goals without sacrificing performance.

Extreme care with vitamin intake, electrolyte balance, and meal timing is required in the crucial days preceding the battle. To maximize recuperation and treat any possible deficiencies, nutrient-dense meals and supplements should be included. Fighters should perfect their hydration tactics to guarantee they are mentally and physically prepared for battle when they step foot in the ring or cage.

Not only is the combat itself important, but so is the time immediately after it. Essential components of a thorough post-fight nutrition regimen include rehydrating, nutritional restoration, and psychological healing. In order to promote long-term health and sustained athletic performance, this phase lays the scene for the future training cycle.

Tailoring one's diet to one's training schedule and fight preparation is an ever-changing and growing process. Athletes require a personalized strategy that takes into account their unique requirements and performance objectives, as well as a sophisticated grasp of nutritional fundamentals. Combatants can improve their physical condition and performance by coordinating their diet with their training and recuperation plans.

Supplements for Fighters

Reaching one's full potential in the rigorous world of combat sports requires a careful integration of structured training with a sophisticated approach to diet. Although a balanced diet is the foundation of a fighter's nutrition, the extreme physical demands of their training frequently call for additional measures to provide complete nutritional support. This article delves into a specialized supplement program designed to meet the unique needs of boxers, with an emphasis on building physical resilience and optimizing performance.

Protein supplements are an essential part of every fighter's supplement routine. These supplements are crucial for speeding recovery after intense workouts since they are known to be essential for muscle development and repair. Among the many post-workout options, whey protein stands out due to its fast absorption and the amino acids it provides, which are vital for starting the healing process. On the other hand, casein protein helps maintain muscle integrity during periods of rest by slowly releasing amino acids, unlike casein.

As a vital component of a fighter's supplementary arsenal, Branched-Chain Amino Acids (BCAAs) round out the protein spectrum. The synthesis of muscle protein is greatly aided by BCAAs, which consist of valine, isoleucine, and leucine. The addition of BCAAs to the routine has many benefits, including reducing muscle fatigue, increasing stamina, and protecting muscular tissue from damage caused by intense exercise. Unlike other types of amino acids, BCAAs can help muscles function even when the body isn't immediately making them.

PART III

WEIGHT MANAGEMENT
STRATEGIES

It takes a holistic and deliberate strategy that includes food and lifestyle decisions to reach and stay at a healthy weight. For those in search of reliable methods of weight loss, the Fighter Diet provides a solid foundation based on the principle of controlled eating. Optimal performance and long-term health are both promoted by switching to a fighter diet.

Maintaining a healthy macronutrient balance is essential to the Fighter Diet approach. Essential for energy production, skeletal muscle development, and metabolic balance, proteins, carbs, and fats are the building blocks of a healthy diet. An efficient and long-lasting diet plan may be developed by precisely adjusting the amounts of these macronutrients. In order to meet energy needs and feel full, it's best to eat a combination of lean proteins, complex carbs, and healthy fats.

A fundamental tenet of the Fighter Diet is calorie restriction, which places an emphasis on eating with awareness and intention. Accurate dietary plan modifications are possible when calorie demands are understood in relation to variables including age, gender, activity level, and fitness objectives. Losing weight healthily and steadily while maintaining muscle mass is possible when people stick to a restricted calorie intake.

The Fighter Diet is structured around carefully planned meal timings that boost performance and metabolism. To maintain steady energy levels and avoid crashes, it's best to eat small, well-balanced meals often throughout the day. In addition, the diet before and after workouts is carefully designed to help with performance, recuperation, and muscle maintenance.

The importance of being hydrated is frequently overlooked, yet it plays a crucial role in managing weight. Staying hydrated helps regulate hunger levels and promotes metabolic processes. Eating meals high in water content and drinking enough of water will help you feel full on fewer calories, which in turn reduces the risk of overeating and improves your health in general.

When used wisely, supplements may supplement the Fighter Diet by filling in any nutritional shortages and improving performance. The selection of supplements should be guided by consultation with healthcare specialists or nutrition experts to ensure they correspond with individual needs and goals.

Incorporating regular physical activity is essential to the Fighter Diet's comprehensive approach to weight management, in addition to food concerns.

To maximize metabolic rate, fat burning, and general body composition, it is best to combine aerobic activity with strength training and flexibility exercises.

The Fighter Diet is an evidence-based and sophisticated strategy for losing weight. Achieving long-term, health-oriented weight loss and optimal physical performance is within reach when people put an emphasis on a balanced diet, calorie restriction, meal timing, adequate hydration, and synergistic supplements.

Mental Toughness and Nutrition

Mental toughness is an essential asset for the committed athlete in the world of competitive sports, where the difference between winning and losing is sometimes hair-thin. When it comes to a fighter's diet in particular, the correlation between mental toughness and nutrition becomes an important consideration in the quest for optimal performance. The complicated web of relationships between the mind and body necessitates a sophisticated comprehension of the ways in which dietary decisions affect mental acuity and performance.

Both the training crucible and the kitchen are important places to build mental resilience. A fighter's diet is an intricate plan that affects their mental and physical sharpness; it's not just a list of macronutrients. The balance of hormones, neurotransmitter activity, and general cognitive ability are all impacted by the food we eat. A solid foundation of optimal nutrition provides the energy and focus needed to overcome the mental hurdles of competition, laying the groundwork for mental resilience.

Whole, nutrient-dense meals are fundamental to the fighter's diet because they support the body and the mind. Vegetables and whole grains are good examples of complex carbs since they provide a constant supply of energy and help maintain the consistent blood sugar levels needed for prolonged mental attention. Amino acid-rich lean proteins help make neurotransmitters, which affect how our brains work. Enhancing cognitive flexibility and resilience in the face of stress, healthy fats like omega-3 fatty acids are included to enhance brain health.

The importance of being hydrated is often underappreciated, although it is crucial for mental acuity. Athletes are particularly vulnerable to the negative effects of dehydration on their performance, which include impaired cognitive function and slower response times. The diligent warrior knows that staying hydrated is the foundation of mental strength.

It is impossible to exaggerate the mental and emotional benefits of a regimented fighter's diet in addition to its obvious physiological advantages. Consistently following a diet plan is similar to the mental toughness needed to succeed in a competitive setting. A mindset of dedication, perseverance, and control is fostered by deliberate culinary decisions; these traits carry over into the arena and beyond.

One of the most important factors in achieving success in combat sports is the complementary nature of mental toughness and proper nutrition. The comprehensive approach needed for top performance is shown by a fighter's diet, which is carefully crafted to fuel the body and mind. Athletes may achieve their mental and physical potential by understanding the connection between nutrition and resilience, and by doing so, they will be better prepared to win in and out of the ring.

Overcoming Challenges and Adversities in Your Fighter Diet Journey

Setting off on a fighter diet path is an arduous endeavor that calls for mental fortitude to persevere through hardships and obstacles as well as physical strength. Recognizing and resolving challenges is essential for long-term success in the discipline-intensive field of nutrition and fitness.

Overcoming the urge to eat poorly is one of the biggest obstacles that people encounter on their road to a fighter diet. Nowadays, we're inundated with fast food joints selling processed foods that might not be the healthiest choice for a fighter's diet. A well-thought-out strategy, including careful meal planning and the development of self-control to avoid cravings, is necessary to overcome this obstacle.

The fact that life is full of surprises, which can throw off long-established habits, is another obstacle. Staying true to the warrior diet principles in the face of challenges like hectic work schedules, unforeseen events, or family duties calls for flexibility and a proactive attitude. To overcome these obstacles without halting development, it is helpful to plan ahead and be flexible with one's diet.

It would be a disservice to the fighter diet journey's mental component to ignore it. It can be challenging to stay motivated, particularly when you hit a plateau or see a slowdown in your progress. Athletes and fighters at the professional level stress the need of having a positive outlook on the trip, setting reasonable and attainable objectives, and enjoying even the smallest successes. The mental challenges that come with sticking to a strict diet plan are real, but building a resilient mindset—one that is persistent and compassionate toward oneself—can help tremendously.

Whether it's a cheat meal that you didn't anticipate, a missed workout, or a momentary lack of discipline, setbacks are inevitable. An expert on the fighter diet would see these setbacks as opportunities to grow, adjust their focus as needed, and keep going even when things become tough. The capacity to recover more quickly and with more strength from setbacks is what really defines resilience, not the absence of hardship.

There are many obstacles along the way of a fighter diet, but there are also many opportunities for personal development and progress. Individuals may triumph over the challenges they face on their path to health and fitness optimisation by adopting a professional mentality that incorporates strategic preparation, flexibility, and mental resilience.

Recovery Protocols: From Ice Baths to Sleep Hygiene

For optimal performance and optimum physical condition, recovery must be a part of every fighter's training and nutrition plan. Incorporating a thorough set of recovery routines, including sleep hygiene and ice baths, may greatly improve an athlete's capacity to recover from strenuous workouts and reduce the likelihood of injuries.

The combat sports community has recently given ice baths the attention they deserve as a tried-and-true method of recuperation. By narrowing blood vessels and easing waste product evacuation from the damaged tissues, low temperatures can reduce inflammation and muscular pain. To speed up recovery and get the body ready for training, fighters should use ice baths in their recovery regimen on a regular basis.

The frequently-overlooked but fundamental component of rehabilitation is proper sleep hygiene, which is just as important. The body's ability to repair and regenerate depends on getting a good night's sleep, which is essential for things like muscle recovery and general health. The cornerstones of good sleep hygiene for a fighter are a regular sleep schedule, an ideal sleeping environment, and the prioritization of sufficient sleep length. In addition to aiding in physical healing, these techniques also improve mental clarity, which is crucial for fighters to keep their attention and sharpness up throughout intense training.

An essential component of successful recovery, hydration is frequently disregarded in recovery conversations. Keeping yourself properly hydrated is essential before, during, and after strenuous physical activity because it helps the body carry nutrients, eliminate waste, and control temperature. It is crucial for fighters to drink enough of water, refill their electrolytes as needed, and strategically organize their hydration according to their training and competition schedules in order to keep their fluid balance ideal.

A fighter's rehabilitation path isn't complete without nutritional tactics. Protein aids in muscle recovery, while carbs restore glycogen reserves; a balanced combination of macronutrients is ideal for post-workout meals. Under the supervision of a trained nutritionist, customized supplements can also aid in recovery by meeting individual demands while also improving general health.

A fighter's dedication to healing goes beyond what happens on the training mat and in the kitchen. Fighters can develop a comprehensive strategy for recovery by combining several regimens, including as ice baths, sleep hygiene, hydration, and diet. The fighters are prepared to confront the mental and physical obstacles that come with their hard pursuits thanks to this all-encompassing method, which strengthens both their physical and mental resilience.

Integrating Mindfulness and Stress Management for Peak Performance

A fighter's eating regimen must incorporate mindfulness practices and stress management techniques in order to achieve prolonged top performance, acknowledging the complex relationship between the mind and body.

Combatants looking to fortify their mental fortitude might benefit greatly from practicing mindfulness, which has its origins in age-old techniques like meditation and deep breathing. Athletes learn to concentrate better, control their emotions, and overcome the obstacles of demanding training programs by focusing on the here and now. Mindfulness training can help build the mental toughness that is just as important as physical strength for success in the brutal world of combat sports.

Recognizing and reducing the many stresses that come with a fighter's lifestyle is an important part of stress management, which is a cornerstone of peak performance. Unmanaged stress may damage physical health and prevent optimal performance, whether it's from external expectations, demanding training regimens, or the pressure of competition. Combatants may better handle stress by using tried-and-true methods like progressive muscle relaxation, visualizing a positive end, and creating clear goals for themselves.

Mindfulness and stress management go hand in hand because they both help the combatant achieve mental harmony. Proactively practicing mindfulness can help athletes develop resilience and create a mental space that is more receptive to stress management. In contrast, stress management equips combatants with actionable strategies for overcoming the inevitable obstacles that may otherwise throw their mental balance into a loop.

Mindfulness may be applied to the field of nutrition through the practice of mindful eating. In addition to helping combatants optimize their vitamin absorption, teaching them to relish and enjoy every mouthful promotes a healthy connection with food. In addition, practicing relaxation methods before meals can help keep the digestive tract in a calm condition, which improves nutritional absorption.

Incorporating stress management and mindfulness into a fighter's diet is a comprehensive strategy that recognizes the complex interplay between mental and physical health. Athletes can reach a level of peak performance beyond what is possible with a strictly physical approach by focusing on both components. This comprehensive approach exemplifies a fighter's dedication to greatness and longevity in the combat game, where mental resilience is just as important as physical power.

PART IV

DELICIOUSLY SIMPLE RECIPES YOU MUST TRY!

Mango-Ginger Smoothie

<u>Ingredients</u>

½ cup cooked red lentils (see Tips), cooled

1 cup frozen mango chunks

¾ cup carrot juice

1 teaspoon chopped fresh ginger

1 teaspoon honey

Pinch of ground cardamom, plus more for garnish

3 ice cubes

Preparation

Place lentils, mango, carrot juice, ginger, honey, cardamom and ice cubes in a blender. Blend on high until very smooth, 2 to 3 minutes. Garnish with more cardamom, if desired.

Overnight Quinoa Pudding

Ingredients

1 cup cooked and cooled quinoa

¾ cup plain kefir

1 tablespoon chia seeds, plus more for serving

2 teaspoons pure maple syrup

¼ teaspoon vanilla extract

Dash of ground cinnamon

1 cup Fresh berries for serving

Preparation

Combine quinoa, kefir, chia seeds, maple syrup, vanilla and cinnamon in a bowl or jar. Refrigerate overnight. To serve, top with berries and more chia, if desired.

Chocolate-Banana Overnight Oats

Ingredients

½ cup old-fashioned rolled oats (see Tip)

½ cup water

Pinch of salt

½ small banana, sliced

1 tablespoon chocolate-hazelnut spread

Pinch of flaky sea salt

Preparation

Combine oats, water and salt in a jar or bowl and stir. Cover and refrigerate overnight.

In the morning, heat the oats, if desired, or eat cold. Top with banana, chocolate-hazelnut spread and sea salt.

Overnight Oats with Chia Seeds

Ingredients

1 ⅓ cups unsweetened plain almond milk

1 cup old-fashioned rolled oats

¼ cup low-fat plain strained yogurt (such as Greek-style)

1 tablespoon chia seeds

¼ teaspoon ground cinnamon

⅛ teaspoon salt

¾ cup chopped peaches, thawed if frozen, divided

¼ cup chopped pecans plus 2 tablespoons, divided

Pure maple syrup for serving (optional)

Preparation

Combine almond milk, oats, yogurt, chia seeds, cinnamon, salt, 1/2 cup peaches and 1/4 cup pecans in a medium bowl; stir to mix well. Cover and refrigerate until the oats have absorbed the liquid and the mixture has thickened, at least 8 hours or up to 5 days.

Divide the oats between 2 bowls. Top each bowl with 2 tablespoons peaches and 1 tablespoon pecans. Drizzle with maple syrup, if desired.

Tofu & Vegetable Scramble

Ingredients

1 ½ teaspoons extra-virgin olive oil

5 ounces extra-firm tofu, drained and cubed

1 cup chopped vegetables, such as zucchini, mushrooms and onions

½ teaspoon spice of choice, such as chili powder or ground cumin

Pinch of ground pepper

⅓ cup canned chickpeas, rinsed

¼ cup pico de gallo or salsa

¼ cup shredded Cheddar cheese, preferably sharp (1 oz.)

1 dash Hot sauce and chopped cilantro to taste

Preparation

Heat oil in a large nonstick skillet over medium-high heat. Add tofu, vegetables, spice and pepper; cook, stirring often, until the vegetables are softened, 5 to 7 minutes.

Add chickpeas and pico de gallo (or salsa) and heat through, 1 to 2 minutes.

Remove from heat, gather the scramble into one section of the pan, top with Cheddar cheese and let melt off the heat. Serve with hot sauce and cilantro, if desired.

Quick Breakfast Taco

Ingredients

2 corn tortillas

1 tablespoon salsa

2 tablespoons shredded reduced-fat Cheddar cheese

½ cup liquid egg substitute, such as Egg Beaters

Preparation

Top tortillas with salsa and cheese. Heat in the microwave until the cheese is melted, about 30 seconds.

Meanwhile coat a small nonstick skillet with cooking spray. Heat over medium heat, add egg substitute and cook, stirring, until the eggs are cooked through, about 90 seconds. Divide the scrambled egg between the tacos.

Egg & Salmon Sandwich

Ingredients

½ teaspoon extra-virgin olive oil

1 tablespoon finely chopped red onion

2 large egg whites, beaten

Pinch of salt

1/2 teaspoon capers, rinsed and chopped (optional)

1 ounce smoked salmon

1 slice tomato

1 whole-wheat English muffin, split and toasted

Preparation

Heat oil in a small nonstick skillet over medium heat. Add onion and cook, stirring, until it begins to soften, about 1 minute. Add egg whites, salt and capers (if using) and cook, stirring constantly, until whites are set, about 30 seconds.

To make the sandwich, layer the egg whites, smoked salmon and tomato on English muffin.

Artichoke & Egg Tartine

<u>Ingredients</u>

1 teaspoon extra-virgin olive oil

½ cup finely chopped thawed frozen artichoke hearts

1 sliced scallion

¼ teaspoon dried oregano

⅛ teaspoon ground pepper

1 slice whole-wheat bread, toasted

2 large eggs, fried or poached

Preparation

Heat oil in a small skillet. Add artichoke hearts, scallion, oregano and pepper; sauté until hot. Spread on toast and top with eggs.

Smoked Trout & Spinach Scrambled Eggs

Ingredients

4 large eggs

2 tablespoons reduced-fat milk

¼ teaspoon ground pepper

Pinch of salt

2 teaspoons grapeseed oil or avocado oil

2 tablespoons finely chopped shallot

½ cup boned and flaked smoked trout (1 1/2 ounces)

1 cup chopped spinach

Preparation

Whisk eggs, milk, pepper and salt in a medium bowl until pale yellow throughout.

Heat oil in a medium nonstick skillet over medium heat. Add shallot and cook, stirring, until starting to brown, 1 to 2 minutes. Add the egg mixture and reduce heat to medium-low. Cook, undisturbed, until the edges start to set, about 30 seconds. Sprinkle trout over the eggs. Using a rubber spatula, gently push and fold the eggs until fluffy and barely set, 2 to 4 minutes. Stir in spinach. Remove from heat, cover and let stand until the spinach is just wilted, 1 to 2 minutes.

Smoked Salmon & Cream Cheese Omelet

Ingredients

2 large eggs

1 teaspoon reduced-fat milk or water

⅛ teaspoon ground pepper, plus more for garnish

Pinch of salt

1 teaspoon butter

2 tablespoons chopped smoked salmon

1 tablespoon cream cheese, softened, or crumbled feta

1 tablespoon finely chopped red onion

1 ½ teaspoons chopped fresh dill, plus more for garnish

<u>Preparation</u>

Whisk eggs, milk (or water), pepper and salt in a small bowl.

Melt butter in a small nonstick skillet over medium-low heat, tilting the pan to make sure the entire bottom is coated. Add the egg mixture and cook for 1 minute without stirring. Sprinkle salmon, cheese, onion and dill over one half of the eggs. Cook for 1 minute. Using a flexible spatula, lift the bare side to let raw egg from the middle flow underneath; you may need to tilt the pan slightly. Continue lifting in different spots until there's almost no raw egg on top. Cook 2 minutes more.

Using the spatula, flip the bare side over the filling, folding the omelet in half, and cook for 1 minute. (If the eggs are starting to brown, lower the heat.) Carefully flip the omelet over and cook 1 minute more. Serve immediately, garnished with more dill and pepper, if desired.

Black Bean & Slaw Bagel

Ingredients

2 cups shredded green cabbage

2 tablespoons chopped fresh cilantro

2 tablespoons lime juice

⅛ teaspoon salt

½ avocado, mashed

1 jalapeño-Cheddar bagel, halved and toasted

1 cup rinsed no-salt-added canned black beans, heated

Preparation
<u>Preparation</u>

Toss cabbage, cilantro, lime juice and salt in a medium bowl. Spread avocado on the top of each bagel half. Top each with 1/2 cup beans and half the slaw.

Chicken Hummus Bowls

Ingredients

1 pound boneless, skinless chicken thighs, trimmed and cut into 1-inch pieces

3 tablespoons extra-virgin olive oil, divided

1 teaspoon ground cumin

1 teaspoon paprika

¼ teaspoon cayenne pepper

¼ teaspoon salt, divided

2 cloves garlic, finely chopped

2 tablespoons lemon juice

2 cups hummus

1 Aleppo pepper, plus more for serving

1 pint cherry tomatoes, halved

¼ cup slivered red onion

¼ cup chopped fresh parsley

Preparation

Position rack in upper third of oven; preheat broiler to high. Line a rimmed baking sheet with foil.

Toss chicken with 1 tablespoon oil, cumin, paprika, cayenne and 1/8 teaspoon salt. Spread evenly on the prepared pan. Broil until just cooked through, 5 to 7 minutes.

Meanwhile, mash garlic and the remaining 1/8 teaspoon salt into a paste with a fork. Transfer to a medium bowl and whisk in lemon juice and the remaining 2 tablespoons oil. Add the chicken and let stand for 5 minutes, stirring occasionally.

Divide hummus among 4 shallow bowls or plates. Top with the chicken and any remaining dressing, cucumber, tomatoes, onion and parsley.

One-Pot Chicken Pesto Pasta with Asparagus

Ingredients

8 ounces whole-wheat penne

1 pound fresh asparagus, trimmed and cut into 2-inch pieces

3 cups shredded cooked chicken breast

1 (7 ounce) container refrigerated basil pesto

1 teaspoon salt

¼ teaspoon ground pepper

1 ounce Parmesan cheese, grated (about 1/4 cup)

Small fresh basil leaves for garnish

Preparation

Cook pasta in a large pot according to package directions. Add asparagus to the pot during the final 2 minutes of cooking time. Drain, reserving 1/2 cup cooking water.

Return the pasta mixture to the pot; stir in chicken, pesto, salt and pepper. Stir in the reserved cooking water, 1 tablespoon at a time, to reach desired consistency. Transfer the mixture to a serving dish; sprinkle with Parmesan and garnish with basil, if desired. Serve immediately.

Cumin Chicken & Chickpea Stew

<u>**Ingredients**</u>

4 cloves garlic, finely chopped

¾ teaspoon salt, divided

¼ cup lemon juice

1 teaspoon ground cumin

1 teaspoon paprika

½ teaspoon ground pepper

1 pound boneless, skinless chicken breasts, trimmed, cut into 1-inch pieces

1 tablespoon extra-virgin olive oil

1 large yellow onion, chopped

1 14-ounce can no-salt-added diced tomatoes

1 15-ounce can chickpeas, rinsed

¼ cup chopped flat-leaf parsley

Preparation

Mash garlic and 1/2 teaspoon salt on a cutting board with the back of a fork until a paste forms. Transfer to a medium bowl and whisk in lemon juice, cumin, paprika and pepper. Add chicken and stir to coat.

Heat oil in a large cast-iron skillet over medium-high heat. Add onion and cook, stirring occasionally, until golden brown, 6 to 8 minutes. Using a slotted spoon, transfer the chicken to the pan (reserve the marinade) and cook, stirring occasionally, until opaque on the outside, about 4 minutes. Add tomatoes with their juice, chickpeas, the reserved marinade and the remaining 1/4 teaspoon salt. Reduce heat to medium and cook, stirring occasionally, until the chicken is cooked through, 5 to 7 minutes more. Serve sprinkled with parsley.

Chicken Salad-Stuffed Avocados

Ingredients

1 pound boneless, skinless chicken breast

⅓ cup low-fat plain Greek yogurt

¼ cup mayonnaise

1 tablespoon chopped fresh tarragon or 1 teaspoon dried

¾ teaspoon salt

½ teaspoon ground pepper

1 cup diced celery

1 cup seedless red grapes, halved (Optional)

¼ cup toasted chopped pecans

2 firm ripe avocados, halved and pitted

Preparation

Place chicken in a large saucepan and add enough water to cover. Bring to a simmer over medium heat. Reduce heat to maintain a simmer, cover and cook until the chicken registers 165 degrees F with an instant-read thermometer, 12 to 15 minutes. Transfer to a cutting board. Let stand until cool enough to handle, then chop or shred. Refrigerate until cold, about 30 minutes.

Combine yogurt, mayonnaise, tarragon, salt and pepper in a large bowl. Add the cold chicken, celery, grapes (if using) and pecans; stir to combine.

To serve, fill each avocado half with about 1/2 cup chicken salad. (Refrigerate the extra chicken salad for up to 3 days.)

Tips

To make ahead: Refrigerate chicken salad (Steps 1-2) for up to 3 days; fill avocados just before serving.

Baked Halibut & Fennel Packets with Chickpea Salad

Ingredients

1 medium bulb fennel, halved, cored and very thinly sliced

½ small shallot, sliced

¼ cup pitted Kalamata olives, halved

1 ¼ pounds halibut fillet, cut into 4 portions

½ teaspoon salt, divided

¼ teaspoon ground pepper, plus more to taste

1 lemon, cut into 4 slices

½ cup dry white wine

1 (15 ounce) can no-salt-added chickpeas, rinsed

½ cup fresh basil leaves, coarsely chopped

½ cup fresh parsley leaves with tender stems, coarsely chopped

1 clove garlic, minced

1 tablespoon lemon juice

1 tablespoon extra-virgin olive oil

⅓ cup grated Parmesan cheese

Preparation

Preheat oven to 425°F. Cut four 15-inch squares of parchment paper and fold each in half. Unfold, then on one side of the fold line, mound 1/4 of the fennel, 1/4 of the shallot and 1 tablespoon olives. Set 1 piece of fish on top and sprinkle with a pinch each of salt and pepper. Lightly squeeze 1 slice of lemon over the fish, then lay it on top. Drizzle 2 tablespoons wine around the vegetables.

Fold the free side of the parchment over the fish and, starting at the top, fold over and pleat the parchment along the open edge all the way to the bottom, creating a sealed packet. Set on a baking sheet. Repeat to make 4 total packets.

Combine chickpeas, basil, parsley, garlic, lemon juice, oil, and the remaining 1/4 teaspoon salt and pepper to taste in a medium bowl; toss to mix well. Stir in cheese.

Bake the fish packets until they are puffed, 11 to 12 minutes. Let stand for 2 to 3 minutes. Set the packets on individual plates and open them carefully at the table. (Caution: The escaping steam will be hot.) Serve with the chickpea salad.

To make ahead

Refrigerate packets (Steps 1-2) for up to 1 day.

Avocado Egg Salad Sandwiches

Ingredients

½ ripe avocado

1 ½ teaspoons lemon juice

1 teaspoon avocado oil

3 hard-boiled eggs, chopped

¼ cup finely chopped celery (about 1 stalk)

1 tablespoon snipped fresh chives

¼ teaspoon salt

⅛ teaspoon ground pepper

4 slices whole-wheat sandwich bread, toasted

2 leaves lettuce

Preparation

Scoop the flesh from the avocado half into a medium bowl. Add lemon juice and oil; mash until mostly smooth. Add chopped eggs, celery, chives, salt and pepper and stir to combine. Divide the mixture between 2 slices of toast. Top each with a piece of lettuce and another slice of toast.

Creamy Pesto Chicken Salad with Greens

Ingredients

1 pound boneless, skinless chicken breast, trimmed

¼ cup pesto

¼ cup low-fat mayonnaise

3 tablespoons finely chopped red onion

2 tablespoons extra-virgin olive oil

2 tablespoons red-wine vinegar

¼ teaspoon salt

¼ teaspoon ground pepper

1 5-ounce package mixed salad greens (about 8 cups)

1 pint grape or cherry tomatoes, halved

<u>Preparation</u>

Place chicken in a medium saucepan and add water to cover by 1 inch. Bring to a boil. Cover, reduce heat to low and simmer gently until no longer pink in the middle, 10 to 15 minutes. Transfer to a clean cutting board; shred into bite-size pieces when cool enough to handle.

Combine pesto, mayonnaise and onion in a medium bowl. Add the chicken and toss to coat. Whisk oil, vinegar, salt and pepper in a large bowl. Add greens and tomatoes and toss to coat. Divide the green salad among 4 plates and top with the chicken salad.

Beet & Shrimp Winter Salad

Ingredients

Salad

2 cups lightly packed arugula

1 cup lightly packed watercress

1 cup cooked beet wedges

½ cup zucchini ribbons (see Tip)

½ cup thinly sliced fennel

½ cup cooked barley

4 ounces cooked, peeled shrimp (see Tip), tails left on if desired

Fennel fronds for garnish

Vinaigrette

2 tablespoons extra-virgin olive oil

1 tablespoon red- or white-wine vinegar

½ teaspoon Dijon mustard

½ teaspoon minced shallot

¼ teaspoon ground pepper

⅛ teaspoon salt

Preparation

Arrange arugula, watercress, beets, zucchini, fennel, barley and shrimp on a large dinner plate.

Whisk oil, vinegar, mustard, shallot, pepper and salt in a small bowl, then drizzle over the salad. Garnish with fennel fronds, if desired.

Tips

To make zucchini ribbons, thinly shave whole zucchini lengthwise with a vegetable peeler.

Go for sustainably raised shrimp. Look for fresh or frozen shrimp certified by an independent agency, such as the Marine Stewardship Council. If you can't find certified shrimp, choose wild-caught shrimp from North America; it's more likely to be sustainably caught.

Give grains a cooldown: To cool grains down quickly, spread them out on a foil-lined baking sheet. The surface area helps speed cooling, while the foil prevents any residual flavors on the pan from seeping in.

Japanese-Inspired Chicken Noodle Soup

Ingredients

2 tablespoons extra-virgin olive oil

1 cup chopped onion

2 large cloves garlic, minced

1 tablespoon minced fresh ginger

8 cups low-sodium chicken broth

2 pounds bone-in chicken breasts, skin removed

3 cups sliced green cabbage

2 cups sliced shiitake or enoki mushrooms

2 cups julienned carrots

1 ¼ teaspoons salt

½ teaspoon ground pepper

3 cups cooked udon noodles or whole-wheat spaghetti

2 tablespoons white miso (see Tip)

Preparation

Heat oil in a large pot over medium heat. Add onion and garlic and cook, stirring occasionally, until softened, 2 to 3 minutes. Add ginger; cook, stirring, for 1 minute. Add broth and chicken. Cover, increase heat to high and bring to a simmer. Uncover and cook, turning the chicken occasionally, until an instant-read thermometer inserted into the thickest part without touching bone registers 165 degrees F, 20 to 22 minutes. Skim any foam from the surface as the chicken cooks. Transfer the chicken to a clean cutting board. When cool enough to handle, remove the meat from the bones and shred.

Meanwhile, add cabbage, mushrooms and carrots to the pot; return to a simmer. Cook until vegetables are tender, 4 to 10 minutes. Stir in the shredded chicken, salt, pepper and noodles and cook until heated through, about 3 minutes more. Remove from heat and stir in miso.

Tips

Tip: Miso is a fermented soybean paste that adds flavor to dishes like soups and sauces. It is available in different colors; in general, the lighter the color, the milder the flavor. Look for miso alongside refrigerated tofu. It keeps in the refrigerator for at least a year.

To make ahead: Cover and refrigerate, without the noodles and miso, for up to 3 days. To serve, stir in noodles and reheat, then stir in miso.

Chicken Quinoa Fried Rice

<u>Ingredients</u>

1 teaspoon peanut oil plus 2 tablespoons, divided

2 large eggs, beaten

3 scallions, thinly sliced

2 teaspoons grated fresh ginger

2 teaspoons minced garlic

1 pound boneless, skinless chicken thighs, trimmed and cut into 1/2-inch pieces

½ cup diced red bell pepper

½ cup diced carrot

½ cup peas, fresh or frozen (thawed)

2 cups cold cooked quinoa

3 tablespoons reduced-sodium tamari or soy sauce

1 teaspoon toasted (dark) sesame oil (Optional)

<u>Preparation</u>

Heat 1 teaspoon oil in a large flat-bottom carbon-steel wok or large heavy skillet over high heat. Add eggs and cook, without stirring, until fully cooked on one side, about 30 seconds. Flip and cook until just cooked through, about 15 seconds. Transfer to a cutting board and cut into 1/2-inch pieces.

Add 1 tablespoon oil to the pan along with scallions, ginger and garlic; cook, stirring, until the scallions have softened, about 30 seconds. Add chicken and cook, stirring, for 1 minute. Add bell pepper, carrot and peas; cook, stirring, until just tender, 2 to 4 minutes. Transfer everything to a large plate.

Add the remaining 1 tablespoon oil to the pan; add quinoa and stir until hot, 1 to 2 minutes. As you stir, pull the quinoa from the bottom to the top so it all gets coated with oil and evenly cooked.

Return the chicken, vegetables and eggs to the pan. Add tamari (or soy sauce) and stir until well combined. Serve drizzled with sesame oil (if using).

Tips

People with celiac disease or gluten-sensitivity should use soy sauces that are labeled "gluten-free," as soy sauce may contain wheat or other gluten-containing sweeteners and flavors.

Skillet Chili Mac

Ingredients

12 ounces whole-wheat elbow noodles, rotini or fusilli

2 tablespoons extra-virgin olive oil

1 large onion, diced

2 medium poblano peppers and/or green bell peppers

1 medium stalk celery, diced

3 cloves garlic, minced

1 pound lean ground beef

3 tablespoons chili powder

½ teaspoon salt

1 (28 ounce) can diced tomatoes

1 cup low-sodium beef broth

1 (15 ounce) can low-sodium kidney beans or chili beans, rinsed

½ cup sour cream

¾ cup shredded sharp Cheddar cheese

Sliced scallions and/or pickled jalapeños for garnish

Preparation

Cook pasta 2 minutes less than the package directions. Drain.

Meanwhile, heat oil in a large skillet over medium-high heat. Add onion, peppers and celery and cook, stirring often, until softened, 4 to 5 minutes. Add garlic and cook, stirring, for 30 seconds. Add beef, chili powder and salt; cook, stirring and breaking up with a spoon, until the beef is no longer pink, 4 to 5 minutes.

Add tomatoes with their juice and broth; bring to a boil over high heat and cook for 2 minutes. Add beans and the pasta, reduce heat to medium and cook, stirring often, until hot, 1 to 2 minutes. Remove from heat. Fold in sour cream. Serve topped with Cheddar and scallions and/or pickled jalapeños, if desired.

Slow-Cooker Buffalo Chicken Chili

<u>Ingredients</u>

1 pound boneless, skinless chicken breast

1 (15 ounce) can no-salt-added black beans, rinsed

1 (15 ounce) can no-salt-added chickpeas, rinsed

1 (15 ounce) can no-salt-added diced tomatoes

1 (15 ounce) can unsalted tomato sauce

½ medium onion, finely chopped

1 cup unsalted chicken broth

⅓ cup Buffalo sauce

2 tablespoons extra-virgin olive oil

½ teaspoon dried oregano

¼ teaspoon garlic powder

¼ cup crumbled blue cheese

¼ cup sour cream (Optional)

<u>Preparation</u>

Combine chicken, beans, chickpeas, tomatoes, tomato sauce, onion, broth, Buffalo sauce, oil, oregano and garlic powder in a 5- to 6-quart slow cooker. Cover and cook on High for 4 hours. Remove the chicken and place on a cutting board. Let cool slightly; roughly shred with two forks and return to the slow cooker. Stir in blue cheese and sour cream, if using.

Equipment

5- to 6-quart slow cooker

Koshari (Egyptian Lentils, Rice & Pasta)

Ingredients

Koshari

1 tablespoon sunflower oil

1 ⅓ cups long-grain brown rice, such as brown basmati

2 teaspoons ground cumin

¾ teaspoon salt

½ teaspoon ground pepper

2 ⅔ cups water

4 ounces whole-wheat spaghetti

1 (15 ounce) can no-salt-added brown lentils, rinsed

1 (15 ounce) can no-salt-added chickpeas, rinsed

Shatta

2 cups diced tomatoes

½ cup chopped onion

2 cloves garlic, sliced

1 tablespoon tomato paste

1 tablespoon distilled white vinegar

6 tablespoons ground cumin

¾ teaspoon salt

½ teaspoon ground pepper

1 ⅓ cups water

1 tablespoon red-wine vinegar

1 teaspoon cayenne pepper

Fried Onions

1 ½ cups sunflower oil

1 cup sliced white onion

2 tablespoons cornstarch

Pinch of salt

Dakka

¾ cup water

3 tablespoons distilled white vinegar

1 teaspoon minced garlic

½ teaspoon ground cumin

½ teaspoon salt

Preparation

To prepare koshari: Heat 1 tablespoon oil in a large saucepan over medium heat. Add rice and cook, stirring, for 1 minute. Add 2 teaspoons cumin, 3/4 teaspoon salt and pepper. Cook, stirring, for 1 minute. Add 2 2/3 cups water and bring to a simmer over high heat. Reduce heat to maintain a simmer, cover and cook until the rice is tender, about 35 minutes. Remove from heat and let stand, covered, for 5 minutes.

Meanwhile, prepare shatta: Combine tomatoes, chopped onion, sliced garlic, tomato paste, 1 tablespoon white vinegar, 6 tablespoons cumin, 3/4 teaspoon salt, pepper and 1 1/3 cups water in a medium saucepan. Bring to a boil over high heat, then reduce heat to maintain a lively simmer. Cook, stirring occasionally, until the sauce is thickened, about 20 minutes. Remove from heat and stir in red-wine vinegar and cayenne.

Bring a small saucepan of water to a boil. Break spaghetti into 1- to 2-inch pieces and cook until just tender, 8 to 10 minutes. Drain.

To prepare fried onions: Heat oil in a large skillet to 350 degrees F. Toss sliced onion with cornstarch in a medium bowl. Add half of the onion to the oil and cook until golden, about 6 minutes. Transfer with a slotted spoon to a plate lined with paper towels. Repeat with the remaining onion. Sprinkle with a pinch of salt.

To prepare dakka: Combine water, white vinegar, minced garlic, cumin and salt in a blender; puree for 1 minute. Transfer to a bowl.

Transfer the shatta (tomato mixture) to the blender and puree until smooth.

Gently stir the spaghetti and lentils into the rice. Serve the koshari topped with chickpeas, the shatta, fried onions and dakka.

Chicken Hummus Bowls

<u>**Ingredients**</u>

1 pound boneless, skinless chicken thighs, trimmed and cut into 1-inch pieces

3 tablespoons extra-virgin olive oil, divided

1 teaspoon ground cumin

1 teaspoon paprika

¼ teaspoon cayenne pepper

¼ teaspoon salt, divided

2 cloves garlic, finely chopped

2 tablespoons lemon juice

2 cups hummus

1 Aleppo pepper, plus more for serving

1 pint cherry tomatoes, halved

¼ cup slivered red onion

¼ cup chopped fresh parsley

<u>Preparation</u>

Position rack in upper third of oven; preheat broiler to high. Line a rimmed baking sheet with foil.

Toss chicken with 1 tablespoon oil, cumin, paprika, cayenne and 1/8 teaspoon salt. Spread evenly on the prepared pan. Broil until just cooked through, 5 to 7 minutes.

Meanwhile, mash garlic and the remaining 1/8 teaspoon salt into a paste with a fork. Transfer to a medium bowl and whisk in lemon juice and the remaining 2 tablespoons oil. Add the chicken and let stand for 5 minutes, stirring occasionally.

Divide hummus among 4 shallow bowls or plates. Top with the chicken and any remaining dressing, cucumber, tomatoes, onion and parsley.

Stuffed Pepper Soup

<u>Ingredients</u>

1 tablespoon extra-virgin olive oil

3 large bell peppers, chopped

1 poblano pepper, chopped

1 medium onion, chopped, plus more for serving

1 pound lean ground beef

2 cloves garlic, minced

2 teaspoons ground cumin

1 teaspoon ground coriander

½ teaspoon ground pepper

¼ teaspoon salt

4 cups low-sodium chicken broth

1 cup quick-cooking brown rice

¼ cup chopped fresh cilantro, plus more for serving

Shredded Cheddar cheese & crushed tortilla chips for serving

<u>Preparation</u>

Heat oil in a large pot over medium-high heat. Add bell peppers, poblano and onion and cook, stirring often, until starting to soften, about 10 minutes. Push the vegetables to the edges. Add beef, garlic, cumin, coriander, ground pepper and salt to the middle and cook, crumbling the beef with a wooden spoon, until it's no longer pink, 3 to 5 minutes.

Stir in broth and rice and bring to a boil. Reduce heat to maintain a low simmer, cover and cook until the rice is tender, 15 to 20 minutes. Remove from heat and stir in cilantro.

Serve the soup topped with cheese, corn chips and more onion and cilantro, if desired.

To make ahead

Refrigerate for up to 3 days.

Garlic-Herb Roast Pork Tenderloin with Parsnip Puree & Kale

Ingredients

1 pound parsnips, peeled and sliced

1 cup whole milk

2 tablespoons unsalted butter

¾ teaspoon salt, divided

¾ teaspoon ground white pepper, divided

1 tablespoon finely chopped fresh rosemary

1 tablespoon finely chopped fresh thyme

3 cloves garlic, minced, divided

1 pound pork tenderloin

2 tablespoons extra-virgin olive oil, divided

10 cups chopped kale

<u>Preparation</u>

Preheat oven to 425°F.

Combine parsnips, milk, butter and 1/4 teaspoon each salt and pepper in a small saucepan. Bring to a simmer, cover and cook until the parsnips are tender, about 15 minutes. Let cool for 5 minutes. Transfer the parsnips and cooking liquid to a food processor and process until smooth. Return the mixture to the pan and cover to keep warm.

Meanwhile, combine rosemary, thyme and 2 cloves garlic on a cutting board. Rub pork with 1 tablespoon oil and roll in the herb mixture. Sprinkle with 1/4 teaspoon each salt and pepper. Heat a large ovenproof skillet over medium-high heat and add the pork. Cook until browned on all sides, about 4 minutes total (adjust heat as necessary to avoid burning the garlic). Transfer the pan to the oven. Roast until the internal temperature of the pork registers 145°F, 12 to 18 minutes. Transfer the pork to a clean cutting board and let rest for 5 minutes.

While the pork rests, add the remaining 1 tablespoon oil to the drippings in the pan (remember, the handle will be hot) and return to medium-high heat. Add kale and cook, stirring occasionally, until just wilted, about 5 minutes. Stir in the remaining 1 clove garlic and 1/4 teaspoon each salt and pepper.

Slice the pork and serve with the parsnip puree and kale.

Chickpea Pasta with Mushrooms & Kale

<u>Ingredients</u>

8 ounces chickpea rotini or penne (see Tip)

¼ cup extra-virgin olive oil

2 large cloves garlic, sliced

Pinch of crushed red pepper

8 cups chopped kale

8 ounces cremini mushrooms, quartered

½ teaspoon dried thyme

½ teaspoon salt

Grated Parmesan cheese for serving (optional)

Preparation

Cook pasta according to package directions. Reserve 1 cup of the cooking water, then drain.

Meanwhile, heat oil in a large skillet over medium heat. Add garlic and crushed red pepper; cook, stirring once, until fragrant, about 1 minute. Add kale, mushrooms, thyme and salt; cook, stirring occasionally, until the vegetables are soft, about 5 minutes.

Stir in the pasta and enough of the reserved water to coat; cook, stirring, until combined and hot, about 1 minute more. Serve topped with Parmesan, if desired.

Tip:

We chose chickpea pasta for this dish instead of whole-wheat because it's packed with tons of fiber, protein and nutrients—some brands provide more than 40% of your daily recommended fiber, plus 20 grams of protein per serving. Look for it with other gluten-free pastas.

Garlic-Anchovy Pasta with Broccolini

Ingredients

2 tablespoons extra-virgin olive oil

6 anchovy fillets (see Tip)

4 cloves garlic, thinly sliced

Pinch of crushed red pepper

1 (5 ounce) package baby spinach

8 ounces whole-wheat angel hair pasta

2 bunches broccolini or 1 bunch broccoli rabe, trimmed and coarsely chopped

¼ cup chopped fresh parsley

¼ teaspoon salt

½ cup chopped almonds, toasted

4 ounces goat cheese, crumbled

Grated lemon zest for garnish

Preparation

Put a large pot of water on to boil.

Meanwhile, heat oil in a large skillet over medium heat. Add anchovies, garlic and crushed red pepper; cook, pressing the anchovies with the back of a wooden spoon to break them up, until fragrant, about 2 minutes. Add spinach in 2 batches and cook, stirring occasionally, until just wilted, about 1 minute. Remove from heat and cover to keep warm.

Add pasta and broccolini (or broccoli rabe) to the boiling water and cook until just tender, 3 to 5 minutes. Reserve 1 cup of the cooking water. Drain and transfer the pasta and vegetables to the skillet; toss to combine, adding enough of the reserved water to achieve desired consistency. Toss with parsley and salt and serve topped with almonds and goat cheese. Garnish with lemon zest, if desired.

Tip:

The little fish that goes a long way, anchovies pack tons of umami flavor into this pasta. Look for packages sporting the blue Marine Stewardship Council certification label for the most sustainable option.

Cajun-Spiced Tofu Tostadas with Beet Crema

Ingredients

8 corn tortillas

2 tablespoons avocado oil, divided

3 cups shredded cabbage

½ mango, julienned (see Tip)

2 tablespoons lime juice, divided

1 tablespoon chopped fresh cilantro

¾ teaspoon salt, divided

1 small cooked beet, shredded

⅓ cup sour cream

1 small clove garlic, grated

1 14- to 16-ounce package extra-firm tofu, drained, crumbled and patted dry

2 tablespoons salt-free Cajun seasoning

1 avocado, diced

Preparation

Position a rack in upper third of oven; preheat to 400°F.

Brush both sides of tortillas with 1 tablespoon oil and arrange on a baking sheet. (It's OK if they overlap a bit; they will shrink as they cook.) Bake, turning once halfway, until browned and very crisp, 10 to 12 minutes. Transfer to a wire rack and let cool.

Meanwhile, toss cabbage, mango, 1 tablespoon lime juice, cilantro and 1/4 teaspoon salt in a medium bowl. Combine beet, sour cream, garlic, the remaining 1 tablespoon lime juice and 1/4 teaspoon salt in a small bowl.

Heat the remaining 1 tablespoon oil in a large cast-iron skillet over medium-high heat. Add tofu, Cajun seasoning and the remaining 1/4 teaspoon salt. Cook, stirring occasionally, until nicely browned, 8 to 10 minutes.

Top the tostadas with the tofu, slaw, beet crema and avocado.

Tip

For flawless julienne pieces, trim a thin slice off the bottom of the mango. Stand it on that end and cut the skin off with a sharp knife. Slice along both sides of the flat pit to yield two large pieces. Turn the pit parallel to you and cut the two smaller pieces of fruit from each side. Thinly slice each piece into long matchsticks.

Maple-Roasted Chicken Thighs with Sweet Potato Wedges and Brussels Sprouts

Ingredients

2 tablespoons pure maple syrup

4 teaspoons olive oil

1 tablespoon snipped fresh thyme

½ teaspoon salt

½ teaspoon black pepper

1 pound sweet potatoes, peeled and cut into 1-inch wedges

1 pound Brussels sprouts, trimmed and halved

Nonstick cooking spray

4 bone-in chicken thighs, skinned

3 tablespoons snipped dried cranberries

3 tablespoons chopped pecans, toasted

<u>Preparation</u>

Preheat oven to 425 degrees F. In a small bowl combine maple syrup, 1 tsp. of the oil, the thyme, 1/4 tsp. of the salt, and 1/4 tsp. of the pepper. In a large bowl combine sweet potatoes and Brussels sprouts. Drizzle with the remaining 1 tbsp. oil and sprinkle with the remaining 1/4 tsp. salt and 1/4 tsp. pepper; toss to coat.

Line a 15x10-inch baking pan with foil. Heat the prepared pan in oven 5 minutes. Remove pan from oven and coat with cooking spray. Arrange chicken, meaty sides down, in center of pan. Arrange vegetables around chicken. Roast 15 minutes.

Turn chicken and vegetables; brush with maple syrup mixture. Roast 15 minutes more or until chicken is done (at least 175 degrees F) and potatoes are tender. Serve topped with pecans and cranberries.

Chicken Club Wraps

Ingredients

1 pound boneless, skinless chicken breast, trimmed

½ teaspoon freshly ground pepper, divided

3 tablespoons nonfat plain Greek yogurt

3 tablespoons cider vinegar

3 tablespoons minced onion

2 tablespoons extra-virgin olive oil

⅛ teaspoon salt

1 medium tomato, chopped

1 avocado, chopped

3 strips cooked bacon, crumbled

8 large leaves red- or green-leaf lettuce

4 10-inch flour tortillas, preferably whole-wheat

<u>**Preparation**</u>

Preheat grill to medium-high.

Sprinkle chicken on both sides with 1/4 teaspoon pepper. Oil the grill grates (see Tip). Grill the chicken, turning once or twice, until an instant-read thermometer inserted into the thickest part registers 165 degrees F, 15 to 18 minutes. Transfer to a clean cutting board and let cool for about 5 minutes.

Meanwhile, whisk yogurt, vinegar, onion, oil, salt and the remaining 1/4 teaspoon pepper in a large bowl. Chop the chicken into bite-size pieces and add to the bowl along with tomato, avocado and bacon; toss to combine.

To assemble the wraps, place 2 lettuce leaves on each tortilla and top with chicken salad (about 1 cup each). Roll up like a burrito. Serve cut in half, if desired.

Vegan Coconut Chickpea Curry

Ingredients

2 teaspoons avocado oil or canola oil

1 cup chopped onion

1 cup diced bell pepper

1 medium zucchini, halved and sliced

1 (15 ounce) can chickpeas, drained and rinsed

1 ½ cups coconut curry simmer sauce (see Tip)

½ cup vegetable broth

4 cups baby spinach

2 cups precooked brown rice, heated according to package instructions

<u>Preparation</u>

Heat oil in a large skillet over medium-high heat. Add onion, pepper and zucchini; cook, stirring often, until the vegetables begin to brown, 5 to 6 minutes.

Add chickpeas, simmer sauce and broth and bring to a simmer, stirring. Reduce heat to medium-low and simmer until the vegetables are tender, 4 to 6 minutes. Stir in spinach just before serving. Serve over rice.

Tips

Tip: Look for a prepared curry sauce with 400 mg sodium or less per serving.

One-Pot Spinach, Chicken Sausage & Feta Pasta

Ingredients

2 tablespoons olive oil

3 links cooked chicken sausage (9 ounces), sliced into rounds

1 cup diced onion (see Tip)

1 clove garlic, minced

1 (8 ounce) can no-salt-added tomato sauce

4 cups lightly packed baby spinach (half of a 5-ounce box)

6 cups cooked whole-wheat rotini pasta

¼ cup chopped pitted Kalamata olives

½ cup finely crumbled feta cheese

¼ cup chopped fresh basil (Optional)

<u>Preparation</u>

Heat oil in a large straight-sided skillet over medium-high heat. Add sausage, onion and garlic; cook, stirring often, until the onion is starting to brown, 4 to 6 minutes. Add tomato sauce, spinach, pasta and olives; cook, stirring often, until bubbling hot and the spinach is wilted, 3 to 5 minutes. Add 1 to 2 tablespoons water, if necessary, to keep the pasta from sticking. Stir in feta and basil, if using.

Easy Pea & Spinach Carbonara

Ingredients

1 ½ tablespoons extra-virgin olive oil

½ cup panko breadcrumbs, preferably whole-wheat

1 small clove garlic, minced

8 tablespoons grated Parmesan cheese, divided

3 tablespoons finely chopped fresh parsley

3 large egg yolks

1 large egg

½ teaspoon ground pepper

¼ teaspoon salt

1 (9 ounce) package fresh tagliatelle or linguine

8 cups baby spinach

1 cup peas (fresh or frozen)

Preparation

Put 10 cups of water in a large pot and bring to a boil over high heat.

Meanwhile, heat oil in a large skillet over medium-high heat. Add breadcrumbs and garlic; cook, stirring frequently, until toasted, about 2 minutes. Transfer to a small bowl and stir in 2 tablespoons Parmesan and parsley. Set aside.

Whisk the remaining 6 tablespoons Parmesan, egg yolks, egg, pepper and salt in a medium bowl.

Cook pasta in the boiling water, stirring occasionally, for 1 minute. Add spinach and peas and cook until the pasta is tender, about 1 minute more. Reserve 1/4 cup of the cooking water. Drain and place in a large bowl.

Slowly whisk the reserved cooking water into the egg mixture. Gradually add the mixture to the pasta, tossing with tongs to combine. Serve topped with the reserved breadcrumb mixture.

Italian Peasant Soup with Cabbage, Beans & Cheese

Ingredients

2 19-ounce or 15-1/2-ounce cans cannellini beans, rinsed, divided

3 tablespoons extra-virgin olive oil, divided

1 medium onion, halved and sliced

4 cups shredded Savoy cabbage, (1/2 medium head)

3 cloves garlic, minced, plus 1 clove garlic, halved

3 14-1/2-ounce can reduced-sodium chicken broth, or 5 1/4 cups vegetable broth

Freshly ground pepper, to taste

8 1/2-inch-thick slices day-old whole-wheat country bread

1 cup grated fontina cheese, or 1/2 cup Parmesan cheese

Preparation

Mash 1 1/2 cups beans with a fork.

Heat 1 teaspoon oil over medium heat in a Dutch oven or soup pot. Add onion and cook, stirring often, until softened and lightly browned, 2 to 3 minutes. Add cabbage and minced garlic; cook, stirring often, until the cabbage has wilted, 2 to 3 minutes. Add broth, mashed beans and whole beans; bring to a simmer. Reduce heat to medium-low, partially cover and simmer until the cabbage is tender, 10 to 12 minutes. Season with pepper.

Shortly before the soup is ready, toast bread lightly and rub with the cut side of the garlic clove (lightly or heavily depending on taste). Divide toast among 8 soup plates. Ladle soup over the toast and sprinkle with cheese. Drizzle about 1 teaspoon oil over each serving. Serve immediately.

Smoky Black Bean & Pepper Soup

Ingredients

2 ½ cups dry black beans, soaked for 8 hours or overnight

2 medium yellow onions

2 medium green bell peppers

1 smoked ham hock (1 1/4 pounds)

2 bay leaves

8 cups water

2 tablespoons extra-virgin olive oil

4 cloves garlic, minced

1 Cubanelle or jalapeño pepper (see Tip), seeded and finely chopped

1 teaspoon ground cumin

1 teaspoon dried oregano

¾ teaspoon salt

1 tablespoon white-wine vinegar or cider vinegar

Roasted red peppers, jalapeño, avocado, red onion & lime wedges for garnish

Preparation

Drain and rinse beans. Finely chop 1 onion and half of the second and set aside. Finely chop 1 bell pepper and set aside. Cut the other into quarters.

Combine the beans, the remaining half onion, the quartered bell pepper, ham hock, bay leaves and water in a pot. Bring to a boil over high heat. Reduce heat to a simmer, cover and cook until the beans are tender, about 1 1/2 hours.

Transfer the ham hock to a clean cutting board and let cool. Discard the onion, bell pepper and bay leaves. Transfer 1 cup of the beans to a small bowl and mash with a fork. Remove the meat from the ham hock and chop.

Heat oil in a large skillet over medium-high heat. Add garlic and cook until fragrant, about 30 seconds. Add Cubanelle (or jalapeno) and the reserved chopped onions and bell pepper. Cook, stirring occasionally, until the vegetables are tender, about 4 minutes. Add cumin, oregano and salt; cook, stirring, for 1 minute. Add vinegar, scraping up any browned bits. Add the mashed beans and cook for 1 minute. 5. Add the vegetables and ham to the beans in the pot. Heat over medium heat, stirring, until hot, about 5 minutes. Serve topped with roasted red peppers, jalapeno, avocado, red onion and lime wedges, if desired.

Slow-Cooker Chicken & Chickpea Soup

<u>Ingredients</u>

1 ½ cups dried chickpeas, soaked overnight

4 cups water

1 large yellow onion, finely chopped

1 (15 ounce) can no-salt-added diced tomatoes, preferably fire-roasted

2 tablespoons tomato paste

4 cloves garlic, finely chopped

1 bay leaf

4 teaspoons ground cumin

4 teaspoons paprika

¼ teaspoon cayenne pepper

¼ teaspoon ground pepper

2 pounds bone-in chicken thighs, skin removed, trimmed

1 (14 ounce) can artichoke hearts, drained and quartered

¼ cup halved pitted oil-cured olives

½ teaspoon salt

¼ cup chopped fresh parsley or cilantro

<u>Preparation</u>

Drain chickpeas and place in a 6-quart or larger slow cooker. Add water, onion, tomatoes and their juice, tomato paste, garlic, bay leaf, cumin, paprika, cayenne and pepper; stir to combine. Add . Cover and cook on Low for 8 hours or High for 4 hours.

Transfer the chicken to a clean cutting board and let cool slightly. Discard bay leaf. Add artichokes, olives and salt to the slow cooker and stir to combine.

Shred the chicken, discarding bones. Stir the chicken into the soup. Serve topped with parsley (or cilantro).

Swedish Yellow Split Pea Soup with Ham

Ingredients

3 cups yellow split peas (about 1 1/2 pounds)

4 cups reduced-sodium chicken broth

4 cups water

2 cups diced yellow onion

1 cup diced carrot

1 cup finely diced celery

8 ounces ham, trimmed and diced

1 tablespoon minced fresh ginger

1 teaspoon dried marjoram

Freshly ground pepper to taste

<u>Preparation</u>

Place split peas in a medium bowl. Wash with cold water until the water runs clear; drain and spread in a 5- to 6-quart slow cooker.

Add broth, water, onion, carrot, celery, ham, ginger and marjoram to the slow cooker (see Tip). Stir to combine.

Cover and cook for 5 hours on High or 7 to 8 hours on Low. Season with pepper.

Tips

Tip: For easy cleanup, try a slow-cooker liner. These heat-resistant, disposable liners fit neatly inside the insert and help prevent food from sticking to the bottom and sides of your slow cooker.

To make ahead: Prep carrots, celery, ginger and dice ham; refrigerate in separate containers.

Winter Vegetable Dal

Ingredients

2 tablespoons coconut oil or canola oil

1 teaspoon brown mustard seeds

1 teaspoon cumin seeds

12 fresh curry leaves (see Tip) or 1 large bay leaf

1 medium onion, finely chopped

1 serrano chile, finely diced

3 tablespoons finely chopped fresh ginger

4 medium cloves garlic, finely chopped

4 ½ cups water

1 ½ cups red lentils (see Tip), rinsed

1 (14 ounce) can "lite" coconut milk

1 ½ teaspoons salt

1 teaspoon ground turmeric

2 ½ cups cubed peeled butternut squash

2 cups cauliflower florets (1-inch)

1 large Yukon Gold potato (about 8 ounces), cut into 1/2-inch chunks

1 teaspoon garam masala

2 tablespoons lime juice

Preparation

Heat oil over medium-high heat in a large pot. Add mustard seeds, cumin seeds and curry leaves (if using) and cook until the seeds begin to pop, about 20 seconds. Add onion, chile, ginger and garlic and cook, stirring occasionally, until the onion is starting to brown, about 5 minutes.

Add bay leaf (if using), water, lentils, coconut milk, salt and turmeric to the pot. Bring to a boil, stirring frequently to make sure the lentils don't stick to the bottom. Add squash, cauliflower and potato; return to a boil. Reduce heat to a simmer and cook, uncovered, stirring occasionally, until the vegetables are just tender when pierced with a fork, 20 to 25 minutes.

Remove from heat; stir in garam masala and lime juice.

Red Pea Soup

<u>Ingredients</u>

1 pound dried kidney beans, soaked overnight

5 cups water

4 cups unsalted chicken broth

2 cups finely chopped cooked chicken

½ cup finely chopped scallions (white and green parts)

¼ cup finely chopped celery

2 tablespoons minced garlic

1 tablespoon finely chopped flat-leaf parsley

1 teaspoon salt

½ teaspoon ground pepper, plus more to taste

½ teaspoon finely chopped fresh thyme leaves

3 tablespoons minced sweet onion, such as Vidalia

Preparation

Drain beans. Place in a large pot along with water, broth, chicken, scallions, celery, garlic, parsley, salt, pepper and thyme. Cover and bring to a boil over high heat; boil for 30 minutes. Reduce heat to a simmer and cook, stirring occasionally, until the beans are tender, about 1 hour. (Add water or broth if the soup seems too thick.)

Season the soup with more pepper, if desired. Ladle into bowls and garnish with sweet onion.

Sichuan Ramen Cup of Noodles with Cabbage & Tofu

Ingredients

6 teaspoons Sichuan chile-bean sauce (toban djan) or chile-garlic sauce

6 teaspoons tahini

1 ½ teaspoons reduced-sodium vegetable bouillon paste (see Tip)

1 ½ teaspoons Chinese rice wine

1 ½ teaspoons packed light brown sugar

¾ teaspoon black vinegar (see Tip)

3 cups shredded napa cabbage

9 ounces extra-firm tofu, cut into 1/2-inch cubes (about 1 1/2 heaping cups)

¾ teaspoon Sichuan peppercorns, coarsely ground

1 ½ cups cooked black or brown rice ramen noodles (see Tip)

1 ½ teaspoons toasted sesame seeds

3 cups very hot water, divided

<u>Preparation</u>

Add 2 teaspoons each chile-bean sauce (or chile-garlic sauce) and tahini, 1/2 teaspoon each bouillon paste, rice wine and brown sugar and 1/4 teaspoon vinegar to each of three 1 1/2-pint canning jars. Layer 1 cup cabbage, 3 ounces tofu (about 1/2 cup), 1/4 teaspoon ground peppercorns and 1/2 cup ramen noodles into each jar. Top each with 1/2 teaspoon sesame seeds. Cover and refrigerate for up to 3 days.

To prepare each jar: Add 1 cup very hot water to the jar, cover and shake until the seasonings are dissolved. Uncover and microwave on High in 1-minute increments until steaming hot, 2 to 3 minutes. Stir well. Let stand a few minutes before eating.

Tips

Tips: Great for flavoring soups, stews and sauces, bouillon paste has a spoonable consistency that makes it easy to portion just the amount you need. To keep sodium in check, opt for reduced-sodium offerings.

For 1 1/2 cups cooked noodles, start with 3 to 4 ounces dry. Boil the noodles about 1 minute less than the package directions so they are slightly underdone. Drain and rinse well with cold water before assembling in jars.

Black vinegar--or ching-kiang vinegar--adds a rich, smoky flavor to many Chinese dishes. Look for it in Asian markets and specialty food shops. Balsamic, sherry or white vinegars can be used as substitutes.

To make ahead: Prepare through Step 1. Refrigerate covered jars for up to 3 days.

Equipment: Three 1 1/2-pint wide-mouth canning jars

Easy Chipotle Chili

<u>Ingredients</u>

2 cups unsalted vegetable broth

1 (15 ounce) can no-salt-added crushed tomatoes

1 cup reduced-sodium vegetarian refried beans

½ cup red enchilada sauce

1 tablespoon chopped chipotle pepper in adobo

1 (15 ounce) can no-salt-added kidney beans, rinsed

1 (15 ounce) can no-salt-added black beans, rinsed

2 (10 ounce) bags frozen mixed vegetables

1 (10 ounce) bag frozen corn

1 teaspoon garlic powder

1 teaspoon onion powder

¾ teaspoon salt

½ cup fresh cilantro, chopped

1 tablespoon cider vinegar

Preparation

Whisk broth, crushed tomatoes, refried beans, enchilada sauce and chipotle together in a large pot. Add kidney beans, black beans, frozen mixed vegetables, frozen corn, garlic powder, onion powder and salt; stir to combine. Bring to a boil over high heat. Reduce heat to medium; cook, stirring occasionally, until the chili has thickened slightly, 12 to 15 minutes.

Remove from heat, stir in cilantro and vinegar.

Slow-Cooker Split Pea Soup with Garlicky Croutons

Ingredients

2 tablespoons olive oil

6 ounces diced ham

1 ½ cups chopped yellow onions (from 1 onion)

1 cup chopped carrots (from 1 carrot)

½ cup chopped celery (from 1 celery stalk)

2 tablespoons minced garlic (about 6 garlic cloves)

½ teaspoon black pepper

6 cups unsalted chicken stock

1 pound dried split peas

1 cup chopped peeled russet potato (from 1 potato)

1 teaspoon kosher salt

1 ½ teaspoons fresh thyme leaves

4 ounces French bread, cut into 1/2-inch slices

<u>Preparation</u>

Heat 1 tablespoon of the oil in a large nonstick skillet over medium-high. Add the ham, onions, carrots, celery, 1 tablespoon of the garlic, and 1/4 teaspoon of the pepper; cook, stirring often, until the mixture is lightly browned and the vegetables are slightly softened, about 10 minutes. Transfer the mixture to a 5- to 6-quart slow cooker.

Stir the stock, split peas, potato, salt, and 3/4 teaspoon of the thyme into the slow cooker. Cover and cook on LOW until the peas are tender, about 8 hours.

Meanwhile, preheat the oven to 350 degrees F. Toss the bread cubes with the remaining 1 tablespoon oil, 1 tablespoon garlic, 1/4 teaspoon pepper, and 3/4 teaspoon thyme. Spread the bread cubes on a baking sheet, and bake in the preheated oven until browned and crisp, about 10 minutes, stirring after 5 minutes.

Remove 2 cups of the soup mixture from the slow cooker, and place in a blender. Remove the center piece of the blender lid (to allow steam to escape); secure the lid on the blender. Place a clean towel over the opening in the blender lid (to avoid splatters). Blend until smooth. Stir the pureed mixture into the soup in the slow cooker. Ladle the soup into bowls. Top evenly with the croutons.

Tips

Multicooker Directions: In Step 1, transfer the cooked ham and vegetables to the inner pot of a 6-quart multicooker. In Step 2, stir in the stock, split peas, potato, salt, and 3/4 teaspoon of the thyme. Lock the lid; turn Pressure Valve to "Venting." Cook on SLOW COOK [Normal] until the peas are tender, about 8 hours. Turn off the cooker. Meanwhile, complete Step 3. In Step 4, purée 2 cups of the soup as in Step 4. Stir the puréed mixture into the soup in the pot. Finish Step 4.

Butternut Squash Soup with Avocado & Chickpeas

Ingredients

1 15-ounce can Amy's Light-in-Sodium Butternut Squash Soup

¾ cup canned chickpeas, rinsed

1 tablespoon lime juice

1 teaspoon curry powder

Pinch of salt

2 tablespoons diced avocado

1 tablespoon nonfat plain Greek yogurt

Preparation

Heat soup in a small saucepan with chickpeas, lime juice, curry powder and salt. To serve, top with avocado and yogurt.

Slow-Cooker Borscht

Ingredients

2 tablespoons canola oil

1 (1 1/2 pound) beef brisket, trimmed and cut in
half

2 cups chopped yellow onions (from 2 onions)

2 tablespoons chopped fresh thyme

8 garlic cloves, chopped (about 2 1/2 tablespoons)

1 tablespoon caraway seeds

½ teaspoon crushed red pepper

1 tablespoon unsalted tomato paste

6 cups unsalted beef stock

2 pounds beet, peeled and cubed

1 pound parsnips, peeled and cubed

1 cup rye berries

2 teaspoons kosher salt

4 cups very thinly sliced red cabbage (from 1 [32-ounce] cabbage head)

2 tablespoons red wine vinegar

1 teaspoon black pepper

½ cup reduced-fat sour cream

¼ cup fresh dill fronds

Preparation

Heat the oil in a large skillet over medium-high. Add the brisket pieces, and cook, turning to brown on all sides, about 8 minutes. Place the brisket pieces in a 4- to 6-quart slow cooker. Add the onions, thyme, and garlic to the skillet, and cook, stirring often and scraping to loosen the browned bits from the bottom of the skillet, about 4 minutes. Add the caraway seeds and crushed red pepper; cook 30 seconds. Add the tomato paste and 2 cups of the stock to the skillet; stir to combine, and bring to a boil. Add the onion mixture to the slow cooker. Stir the beets, parsnips, rye berries, salt, and remaining 4 cups stock into the slow cooker. Cover and cook on LOW until the brisket is tender, 7 hours and 30 minutes.

Remove the brisket pieces, and set aside. Add the cabbage and red wine vinegar to the slow cooker; increase the heat to HIGH, and cook, uncovered, just until the cabbage is wilted, about 15 to 20 minutes.

Meanwhile, shred the brisket using 2 forks. Add the shredded brisket and black pepper to the slow cooker, and stir to combine. Ladle the soup into bowls. Top evenly with the sour cream and dill.

Tips

Multicooker Directions: In Step 1, place the browned brisket pieces in the inner pot of a 6-quart multicooker. Continue with Step 1, adding the cooked onion mixture to the pot; stir in the beets, parsnips, rye berries, salt, and remaining 4 cups stock. Lock the lid; turn Pressure Valve to "Venting." Cook on SLOW COOK [Normal] until the brisket is very tender, about 8 hours. Turn off the cooker. In Step 2, remove the brisket pieces; set aside. Add the cabbage and vinegar to the pot. With the lid off, press SAUTÉ [Normal]; cook, uncovered, just until the cabbage is wilted, stirring occasionally. Meanwhile, complete Step 3.

Split Pea Soup with Chorizo

<u>Ingredients</u>

4 cups low-sodium chicken broth

4 cups water

1 pound Yukon Gold potatoes, diced

2 cups yellow split peas

1 large onion, diced

2 large carrots, sliced

6 cloves garlic, finely chopped

1 tablespoon paprika

2 teaspoons dried oregano

¾ teaspoon salt, divided

1 pound fresh chorizo

½ teaspoon ground pepper

¼ cup Microgreens or sprouts for garnish

Preparation

Combine broth, water, potatoes, split peas, onion, carrots, garlic, paprika, oregano and 1/2 teaspoon salt in a 5- to 6-quart slow cooker. Cook on High for 4 hours or Low for 8 hours.

A few minutes before serving, remove chorizo from its casing and crumble into a large skillet. Cook over medium heat, stirring and crumbling with a spoon, until cooked through, 3 to 5 minutes. Stir the chorizo into the soup along with pepper and the remaining 1/4 teaspoon salt. Garnish with microgreens (or sprouts), if desired.

Tips

To make ahead: Refrigerate for up to 3 days.

Chicken Soup with Recaito & Potatoes

Ingredients

1 tablespoon extra-virgin olive oil

1 teaspoon ground cumin

4 cups lower-sodium chicken broth

1 (12 ounce) jar recaito cooking base (see Tip)

2 cups cubed scrubbed baby gold or Yukon Gold potatoes (1/2-inch)

1 cup cubed scrubbed carrots (1/2-inch)

1 cup chopped red bell pepper

1 ½ cups shredded rotisserie chicken

1 cup frozen green peas

2 tablespoons fresh lime juice

⅛ teaspoon salt

<u>**Preparation**</u>

Heat oil in a medium Dutch oven over medium heat. Add cumin; cook, stirring often, until fragrant, about 1 minute. Stir in broth and recaito; bring to a boil over high heat. Stir in potatoes, carrots and bell pepper. Reduce heat to medium-low and simmer, stirring occasionally, until the vegetables are just tender, 8 to 10 minutes. Stir in chicken and peas; cook, stirring occasionally, until the chicken and peas are heated through, about 2 minutes. Stir in lime juice and salt.

Tip

Recaito is a green puree typically made with culantro, onions, sweet peppers and garlic. It is commonly found in Puerto Rican cuisine and used as a base in many savory dishes. Store-bought versions of recaito often substitute culantro with cilantro, which is milder in flavor. Find it in the international aisle of major supermarkets.

Winter Minestrone

<u>Ingredients</u>

1 pound uncooked Italian or pork sausage links, cut into 3/4-inch slices

2 ½ cups peeled winter squash, such as butternut squash, cut into 1-inch cubes

1 ½ cups cubed potatoes

2 medium fennel bulbs, trimmed and cut into 1-inch pieces

1 large onion, chopped

2 cloves garlic, minced

1 (15 ounce) can red kidney beans, rinsed and drained

½ teaspoon dried sage, crushed

4 cups chicken broth or vegetable broth

1 cup dry white wine

4 cups chopped kale or fresh spinach

Preparation

In a large skillet, cook the sausage until browned; drain well.

In a 5- to 6-quart slow cooker, place squash, potatoes, fennel, onion, garlic, beans and sage. Top with sausage. Pour broth and wine over all.

Cover and cook on Low for 8 to 10 hours or on High for 4 to 5 hours. Stir in kale (or spinach). Cover and cook 5 minutes more.

Bean & Beef Taco Soup

<u>Ingredients</u>

1 tablespoon olive oil

1 cup chopped yellow onion (from 1 medium onion)

¾ cup chopped poblano chile (about 1 medium chile)

1 pound 93/7 lean ground beef sirloin

1 tablespoon minced garlic (about 3 medium garlic cloves)

1 teaspoon ancho chile powder

1 teaspoon ground cumin

½ teaspoon dried oregano

¼ teaspoon cayenne pepper

1 (15 ounce) can no-salt-added tomato sauce

1 (15 ounce) can no-salt-added pinto beans, rinsed and drained

1 (15 ounce) can no-salt-added black beans, rinsed and drained

1 (10 ounce) can diced tomatoes and green chiles (such as Rotel)

1 ½ cups unsalted beef broth

1 cup fresh or frozen (and thawed) corn kernels

¾ teaspoon kosher salt

⅓ cup chopped fresh cilantro, plus more for garnish

1 medium ripe avocado, cut into small cubes

¾ cup tortilla strips (about 1 ounce)

½ cup sour cream

2 ounces pre-shredded Mexican cheese blend (about 1/2 cup)

Lime wedges

Preparation

Heat oil in a large saucepan over medium-high. Add onion and poblano; cook, stirring often, until lightly browned, about 6 minutes. Add ground beef; cook, stirring to crumble, until no longer pink, about 7 minutes. Add garlic, ancho chile powder, cumin, oregano and cayenne; cook, stirring constantly, until fragrant, about 1 minute. Add tomato sauce, pinto and black beans, diced tomatoes, broth, corn and salt; bring to a boil over medium-high. Reduce heat to medium; simmer, undisturbed, about 10 minutes. Remove from heat; stir in cilantro. Top evenly with avocado, tortilla strips, sour cream and cheese. Serve alongside lime wedges.